My Afro Hair, My True Identity

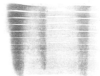

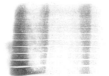

My Afro Hair, My True Identity

A Healthier Way to Grow and Care for Afro Hair

Jane Ezuruike

ISBN: 9780578328942

I thank the Almighty God for the knowledge, wisdom, and understanding He gave me through Jesus Christ to write this book.

To my mom, thanks for your support and encouragement.

CONTENTS

Important Terms to Know

Scalp hair: the hair that grows on the scalp.

Scalp: the skin covering the top of the head.

Hair strand: a single hair.

Hair shaft: the hair that is evident on the scalp.

Hair bulb: the bulb-shaped part of the base of the hair.

Hair root: the farthest part of the hair that is implanted in the hair follicle.

Hair follicle: a structure in the outer layer of the skin that is responsible for hair growth, hair texture, and hair color.

Sebum: the natural oil that moisturizes and nourishes the hair and skin.

Sebaceous gland: the gland that produces sebum.

Chapter One

Intro to Afro Hair

Afro hair is the natural hair type that most people of African descent have. It is a unique type of hair with tightly curled hair strands that vary among individuals. Because of the tight curly feature of Afro hair, it requires a sufficient supply of sebum, the natural oil that keeps the hair and skin moisturized, to travel from the hair root to the tip of the hair strands.

Sebum travels in a helical manner to moisturize Afro hair. This distinctive moisturizing process is one of the major factors that makes Afro hair susceptible to dryness and easy breakage. It is faster for sebum to moisturize the hair from the root to the tip when it moves in a straight pattern. However, it moves in a curly pattern in Afro hair, which is why it takes a little longer to completely lubricate the hair strands.

Afro hair gradually dries-out and becomes hard to style when it does not get sufficient supply of natural oil. This discourages most people from growing their natural hair and makes them resort to chemical and mechanical hair straightening, which are harmful to the hair.

Relying on harmful haircare practices to achieve desired hairstyles is unhealthy. They can lead to hair follicle damage, hair thinning, low hair length retention, and other hair problems. Chemical hair relaxing, for example, might have a link to cancer and uterine fibroids.

Afro hair is truly special and beautiful. If you figure out the right ways to care for your Afro hair and use them, you will get results that will make you fall deeply in love with your natural hair. This applies to all Afro hair types. It does not matter if you have thick or thin hair, if you have tough or soft hair, if you are old or young, or if you are a male or female. Gaining the right knowledge on how to care for your hair will help you grow healthy Afro hair.

It is important to note that attractive hair does not necessarily mean healthy hair. People use harmful haircare methods and products to enhance the appearance of their hair for instant gratification, which leads to serious hair damage in most cases. Do not let the appearance of other people's hair make you look down on your own hair. Growing Afro hair requires patience. If you keep taking the right haircare steps, your hair will continue to grow, stay strong, and be healthy.

The haircare tips shared in this book will be helpful to people with Afro hair, people with different hair types who adopted or plan to adopt children with Afro hair, parents of kids with Afro hair, and anyone who wants to know more about haircare.

As you read along, you will learn how to make close observations to determine when hair products or haircare routines are working or not working for you. You will also learn how using the right hair products, doing the right hairstyles, and taking proper care of your body play huge roles in keeping your hair healthy.

Chapter Two

Afro Haircare Products

Have you ever imagined what life would be like without having access to the real foods your body recognizes? Foods that you need to eat to be healthy. That life is comparable to how Afro hair turns out when the wrong products are consistently being applied to it.

Afro hair thrives the most when hair products made with 100% natural and non-toxic ingredients are used to care for it. The regular hair products on the market, even some of the ones specifically made for Afro hair, are not as safe and effective as they are being advertised.

It might seem like they are working in the early stage of use but using them long-term leads to hair damage. Most of them have ingredients that slightly loosen Afro curl patterns, which becomes a problem later because of the denatured hair structure.

Know that Afro haircare products do not yield the same results for all Afro hair types. The product that works for one person's Afro hair might not work for another person's hair. This being the case, it is important to closely observe the effects of the hair products you apply to know the ones that are working and those that are not working for your hair.

Note how your hair turns out after applying a hair product. Does it stay moisturized or dry-out easily? Does it become brittle and break easily? Does it recoil unevenly? These are some of the variables you always need to watch out for whenever you use a hair product. If you notice consistent undesirable changes after using a product, that probably means the product is not suitable for your hair.

It is advisable to keep the combination at which you use different hair products simple. The simplicity makes it easier for you to know the products that are working for your hair and those causing damage to it. You do not need to spend too much money on haircare products because the health of your hair does not solely rely on the products you apply to it. It also relies on the nourishment it naturally gets from your body.

Be careful when choosing haircare products. Before buying a product, make sure you check the ingredients. If a hair product has an ingredient that does not work for your hair or you do not know, it is better not to buy that product regardless of how it is being marketed. If you are unsure of a specific ingredient in a product but still want to purchase it, you can ask questions to find out the potential benefits and risks of using it before buying.

Checking the ingredients in haircare products before buying or applying them to your hair is what you always need to do because Afro hair is overly sensitive to harmful ingredients.

Hair Moisturizers

Hair moisturizers help with lubricating Afro hair; however, that does not change the fact that sebum is the primary moisturizer your hair needs to stay protected and healthy. Hair moisturizers also protect the hair from the direct effects of harmful environmental agents like germs from polluted air and chemicals used in water treatments.

The commonly used natural hair moisturizers include olive oil, shea butter, castor oil, etc. The best way to find a moisturizer that is suitable for your hair is to try out different natural hair moisturizers, one at a time, and then choose the one that works best for your hair. For example, you can use shea butter for the first few days of your trial and use castor oil days later; then you compare and choose the one that moisturizes your hair better. When Afro hair is moisturized, it is soft, strong, bouncy, shiny, and easy to style.

Be aware that it is possible for products that once worked for your hair to become less effective. This usually happens when they get contaminated or are not original. Your hair can reject these products through showing signs like hair dryness, hair tangling, hair brittleness, and so on. Whenever you notice any of these changes and confirm that a product is not safe for your hair, stop using that product and try other natural products, as directed earlier, to find the one that works best for the current state of your hair.

Different life events can put you in a position where you must change your hair products. For example, if you move to a new place where the water that gets supplied to your home is contaminated, the best thing to do is to switch to more enriched hair products with tougher protective properties to protect your hair. Using the contaminated water to wash your hair without additional hair protective measures can lead to hair dryness, hair weakening, hair discoloration, and other hair problems. You can link these changes to other factors like age or genes without knowing they are connected to the water you are using to wash your hair.

When you find the right hair moisturizer that suits your hair, always apply it after you wash your hair with a hair shampoo. However, refrain from applying excessive amounts of hair moisturizers to your hair as that can interfere with the moisturizing effects of sebum.

Hair Shampoo

It is not easy to find a good natural hair shampoo for Afro hair. As discussed earlier, most of the ones sold in stores are not recommendable because of the chemical additives in them. If you check the labels of these shampoos, you will find out that they contain ingredients that are not safe for your Afro hair. These types of shampoos make your hair to become dry and brittle. The best way to tackle this issue is to learn how to make your own hair shampoo that will not be harmful to your hair.

You can make hair shampoos with African black soap. African black soap is a brownish-black soap made with natural ingredients that are healthy for Afro hair. It is mostly handmade in African countries like Ghana and Nigeria, hence the name. It is easy to make a hair shampoo with African black soap, and it works well when used to wash Afro hair. Black soap shampoo gently cleanses the hair and keeps it moisturized. It lathers well and makes hair washing easier and smoother. You can wash your hair with it regularly without losing your hair's natural oil.

How to Make African Black Soap Shampoo

- Cut out small chunks of black soap and put them in a container with water, preferably warm water. The water should be above the soap level depending on the amount of shampoo you want to make.
- Leave them to dissolve for few minutes or hours.
- Gently filter the dissolved liquid soap with a clean cloth, paper towel, or any permeable material and discard the undissolved particles.
- Use the filtered black soap shampoo to wash your hair.

African black soap is good for the skin, which is another spectacular thing about it. You do not have to worry about it getting on your face or body while washing your hair since it is a medicinal bath soap. It has been used for decades to cure various kinds of skin conditions like acne, ringworm, eczema, etc. Be careful when buying African black soap as some of them are not well prepared. Original African black soap has an earthy smell with no chemical additives in it.

To maintain healthy Afro hair, it is critical to avoid applying any kind of chemical products to your hair. Do not be tempted to relax or texturize your hair for any reason. The chemicals used in making hair relaxers and texturizers are harmful. They can burn your scalp and leave open wounds that lead to hair follicle infections.

Hair dyes are also harmful to the hair and need to be avoided. Applying them might not seem bad, in the initial stage, but they can make you hair too tough and hard to maintain with time. Do not opt for these products because others are using them if you really want your hair to be healthy. When your hair gets damaged from washing it with dirty water, for instance, it can easily bounce back to a healthy state when you stop using the dirty water; but when it is a case of chemical damage, it might not recover. It is better to avoid the stress and be patient with caring for your hair with good natural products.

Hair Product Contamination

Once your hair product gets contaminated, it will no longer be as effective as it is supposed to be for your hair. Instead of helping to keep your hair healthy, it will start stirring up hair problems. Hair product contaminants can chop off your hair like it has been cut with scissors; it is that bad. Always ensure your hair products are not contaminated or expired before you use them. Signs that indicate that a hair product is contaminated include a change in color, smell and consistency of the product, and bad side effects after applying it.

Your hair products can get contaminated in different ways. They can get contaminated if microorganisms get in them or if harmful substances get mixed with them. Always ensure your hair products are properly covered and stored in a clean place. Your products can also get contaminated if germs get transferred from your fingers to them. Make sure your fingers are clean and dry before you use them to take hair products in jar containers.

Chapter Three

When to Wash Your Hair

How often do you wash your hair? People have different opinions on how often Afro hair needs to be washed. Some people wash their hair regularly, while others prefer not to because they believe it leads to hair dryness. It is not hair-washing that causes the hair dryness. Washing Afro hair with the wrong shampoo and contaminated water are the two factors that lead to Afro hair-wash related dryness.

The ingredients used in making regular shampoos strip off needed natural oil from the hair, and contaminants in water can attach to Afro hair strands and restrict the free flow of natural oils through them. If you wash your hair regularly with the right hair shampoo and uncontaminated water, you will not have hair dryness issues after washing your hair.

Afro hair is easier to style when it is clean, and the hairstyles look better when the old products are properly washed off and refreshed with new ones. Regular hair-washing should be included in your haircare routine. You do not need to use a shampoo each time you wash your hair. You can wash your hair with only water sometimes and wash with shampoo when needed. Washing your hair regularly will help keep your scalp clean to avert product buildup, which is one of the factors that make Afro hair difficult to style.

It is so challenging to style Afro hair when it is dirty. Dirt makes it recoil unevenly and applying hair products on top can make it look untidy. The hair products we apply to our hair attract dust and germs. It is important to wash them off regularly and apply fresh ones.

The number of times to wash your hair weekly should depend on the type of environment your hair gets exposed to each day. If you live or work in an environment that harbors dirt or germs, it is advisable to wash your hair every day or every other day to prevent the dirt and germs you were exposed to from building up in your hair.

Germs are opportunistic. If you do not get rid of them once they have gained access to any part of your body, they will establish a territory there and begin to multiply. The replication will then lead to problems like dandruff, ring worm, or other hair infections if your scalp happens to be the affected area.

Dirt makes Afro hair strands susceptible to breakage and tangling, especially the ones in clumps. Clumpy dirt can mat hair strands together and lead to hair breakage when the hair is being combed. Dirt mixed with different types of germs weakens the hair and makes it to break easily. It is more likely for dirty hair with the buildup of germs to suffer serious breakage than clean and freshly moisturized hair.

Dirt also makes the scalp itchy. Scratching your scalp when it is dirty and itchy can result to open wounds that serve as portals of entry for microorganisms to get in your body. This leads to hair infections and other issues that can cause serious problems in the body.

Particles from dirty scalp and hair can get on the face and lead to breakouts. Most facial breakouts are triggered by germs transferred from the hair to the face. Germs can get transferred to the face through scratching a dirty scalp and touching the face with the same hand or from dirty hair to a pillowcase and then to the face during sleep.

In addition to washing your hair regularly, always ensure your comb is clean before using it to comb your hair. Wash your hair combs before and after use to prevent the transfer of germs from them to your hair and scalp.

Water Issues

It is not safe to use treated water to wash your hair. Treated water contains chemicals like chlorine and chloramine, which are harmful to the hair and can build up on the scalp. A possible solution to this issue is to use a water filtration system to filter out contaminants from your water before use. There are different water filtration products on the market today that can help you achieve this goal. Filtered water is worth it and not only good for your hair, but also for drinking, cooking, and brushing your teeth.

You can also boil and filter water to wash your hair. Boiling method is a way of killing microorganisms in water, which can bring it to a safer point to be used to wash the hair. However, the method might not completely remove chemical contaminants from water.

How to Boil and Filter Water for Hair-washing

- Bring your water to a full boil in a clean pot.

- After that, let it cool-off for few minutes to allow the contaminants to settle at the bottom.

- Gently pour the upper part of the water into another clean container and discard the bottom part.

- Filter the drawn water with a clean permeable cloth (or any other good filtration material) into another pot or container.

- Repeat the steps two more times, then allow the final filtered water to cool.

- Pour the water into a bath bucket and gradually take it with a mug to wash your hair.

Note:

You can either wash your hair with the water that runs directly from your shower or use this bucket method. If you prefer to wash your hair while taking a shower, always ensure that you properly wash off the dirt that gets to your body. The residues are usually very sticky and need to be carefully washed off to prevent skin breakouts.

How to Wash Your Afro Hair

- Always put your hair in sections before washing it to reduce hair tangling. It can be in four, five, or more sections depending on the length of your hair. You can hold the sectioned hairs in loose two-strand twists or with loose hair holders. You do not need to section your hair if it is still short.

- After sectioning your hair, run water through it then apply your shampoo.

- Use the shampoo lather to clean your scalp with the tip of your fingers. Do not use your nails to prevent hurting yourself.

- When you feel your scalp is nicely cleaned, proceed to washing your hair, and thoroughly rinse off the shampoo when you are done.

- Detangle your hair by finger detangling or combing with a wide-tooth comb.

- Rinse your hair again to remove shampoo residues.

- Hold back the section you completed in a twist or with a hair holder. Shampoo, rinse, detangle, and hold the other sections the same way. Complete each step from one sectioned hair to another.

- Finally, untwist all the sections and let your hair to air-dry while you put it in a style of your choice.

Note: Two-strand twists are made by twisting two equally sectioned hair strands around each other in a "rope-like twist" from the bottom to the tips.

Additional Points

Run water through your hair while you moisturize it. This makes the detangling and moisturizing process easier and helps with rinsing off most of the contaminants that might have gotten into your moisturizer, so they do not get attached to your hair strands or accumulate on your scalp. It also helps your hair to absorb the moisturizer better. You can use a spray bottle with clean water to moisturize your hair before applying your moisturizer if you are not using the shower method.

Avoid the use of blow dryers and other heat styling tools to groom your hair. They weaken Afro hair shafts, which leads to hair thinning, hair breakage, and low hair retention. Make sure your detangling comb is wide enough without rough teeth. Fine-tooth combs will distort your natural curl pattern. Combs with broken, rough, or sharp teeth, on the other hand, will make your hair break easily if you use them to detangle.

Do not use cotton towels to dry your hair. They soak natural oils from the hair, which leads to hair frizz, hair dryness, and hair breakage. Use soft materials to dry your hair or let it air-dry.

How to Finger Detangle Your Hair

- Moisturize your hair and put it in sections. Separate the sections in twists or any other safer way that works best for you.
- Hold-out one section and gently unravel the twist (if you separated the sections in twists).
- Use one hand to hold the sectioned hair and use the other to gradually detangle your hair strands with your fingers.
- Separate approximately five to ten strands of hair at a time, detangling them from the bottom to the tip until you detangle the hair strands from that section.
- Put the detangled section back in a twist and follow the same steps to detangle the other sections. You

can complete the detangling process while running water through your hair. If you come across matted hair strands, separate them one by one to prevent unnecessary hair breakage.

Hair Washing for Children

When it comes to washing children's hair, you need to make it a routine they look forward to and enjoy. Be gentle when cleaning their scalp and detangling their hair. Just like adults, wash their hair in sections depending on the length and clean their scalps by gently massaging them with the tips of your fingers. You can make the routine fun by singing while telling them why it is important to wash their hair. Use the finger or comb detangling method to detangle their hair after washing.

If your child has Afro hair, but you have a different hair type, keep in mind that your child may start to wonder why his or her hair is different from yours. Once children get to a certain age, they start to question things around them that they do not understand although they might not be verbal about it. It is crucial to find a way to always explain things your children need to know to them.

When it is about hair differences, clearly explain why people have different hair types to them and let them know that all hair types are beautiful. They might not respond, but they can hear and understand you. This helps to protect them from having any mental stress in the process of trying to figure the reasons behind the different hair types.

Always let your children know that their hair type is beautiful. The more you let them know how beautiful their hair is, the more they love their hair, and it will be hard for them to get negatively influenced to alter it in the future.

Chapter Four

Style with Caution

People with Afro hair type do many hairstyles that are unhealthy. These hairstyles lead to all forms of hair damage and low hair length retention that might have led to the assumption that Afro hair hardly grows. Some of these hairstyles are believed to be a part of Afro culture, but they are not fit for your hair and overall well-being.

The common ones include hair braids (done with or without hair extensions), hair threading, wigs, and weaves. Hair braids are usually made tight. It is so rare to find a braided hair that is not tight on the scalp. Some braids are done in such a way that both the skin on the forehead and the hair around the edges are tightly pulled backward. This restricts blood flow to the regions of the head and leads to hair follicle damage, which is one of the reasons people who regularly do braids lose so much hair around their hairline.

Hair threading is a hairstyle you should also avoid as it shares similar negative effects with hair braiding. This hairstyle stretches the hair, which is not favorable for Afro hair. If you stretch your hair a lot, it will lose its ability to evenly recoil back to its natural Afro length. When your hair cannot uniformly recoil back to its natural Afro length, that means it is unhealthy and will require gentle handling to recuperate.

Wigs and weaves are also not safe for your hair. The materials used in making them can cause friction damage to your hair as they rub against each other. The ones done with glues, elastic bands, and tight wig caps interfere with free airflow to the scalp and can lead to poor circulation of blood around the head regions.

Do not let anyone influence you to do these hairstyles. Always remember that not all Afro hair types can withstand the pressures from them. You might embark on the same journey and end up with a serious hair damage, like going bald around your edges, which can take years to regrow.

To better protect your hair, always do loose and low manipulation hairstyles that will not restrain blood flow to any part of your head. Other hair disorders that result from tight hairstyles include:

A. Folliculitis - inflammation of the hair follicles with signs like bumps around hairlines.

B. Stunted hair growth - scars from improperly healed inflamed hair follicles can restrict hair growth.

C. Traction alopecia - the partial or complete absence of hair in an affected area. This is common around the edges.

D. Necrosis - the death of most of the cells around the head due to the lack of blood supply.

E. Inflammation of the lymph nodes - tight hairstyles make the lymph nodes behind the ears and around the neck sore, painful, or prominent.

The best time to style your hair is when it is well moisturized. It is painful to style Afro hair when it is dry, and that increases hair breakage and damage. Know that hair loss and hair breakage are quite different. Hair strands from hair loss cases usually have bulbs attached to their ends, which indicates that the hair was lost from the base of the hair. Hair breakage is the opposite - the broken hair strands do not have bulbs attached to them. Styling your hair when it is moisturized will help reduce the chances of these two hair problems and cause you less pain.

If you notice matted hair strands when styling your hair, gradually untangle the strands one by one. You can spray water to the matted strands to make it easier for you to untangle them. Do not speedily rip them apart to prevent hair breakage.

Hair Trimming

It is essential to trim your hair regularly. Mainly when you notice some strands of your hair growing out so long as to make your curls tangle easily. Regular trimming helps your hair strands stay uniformed, which makes your Afro hair look better when you wear it freely. It also helps to reduce hair tangling and breakage.

It is better to trim your hair when water is running through it. The water helps unlock your hair curls so you can easily detect the uneven hair strands. Always trim in small sections to help keep your hair strands even.

How to Trim Your Afro Hair

▪ Put your hair in small sections.

▪ Hold-out one of the sectioned hairs and align the hair strands properly to ensure that you can see or feel the uneven ones.

▪ Cut off the ends of the uneven hair strands with a pair of sharp scissors. Do not use blunt scissors to prevent any damage to your hair as you struggle to make a cut.

▪ Cut a few inches at a time to avoid cutting off huge chunk of your hair.

▪ Follow the above steps to trim the rest of the sections.

Always put your Afro hair in a loose protective style before going to sleep. Protective styles are hairstyles that keep the hair protected to reduce hair loss and breakage. Protective styles should be loose styles that allow the easy flow of sebum from the root to the tip of your hair strands; if not, the tip of your hair will be at risk of becoming too dry and breaking off easily. You can hold your hair up with a scarf or do loose two-strand twists to keep it protected.

You do not have to do protective styles if your hair is short. Just make sure your hair stays moisturized and cover it with a hair scarf before bed to help retain moisture. You will need to start doing protective styles when your hair grows longer and begins to tangle easily.

How to Style and Wear Your Afro Hair Freely

- Wash, detangle, and hold your hair in loose two-strand twists, as directed earlier.

- Next, gently unravel the twists, one section at a time, and moisturize your hair (if you did not moisturize it before detangling).

- Run water through your hair as you complete these steps.

- Moisturize each section of your hair from the bottom to the tip. Do not put the sectioned hairs back in twists after you moisturize.

- Stop running water through your hair and shake off the excess water at this point.

- Without overly touching or manipulating your hair, use your fingers to gently "even-out" your hair strands to close the gaps that were created while your hair was in sections.

- Finally, allow your hair to air-dry and recoil back to its natural Afro length as it dries.

This hairstyle is easy, painless, and increases hair retention since the hair is styled while it is still wet and moisturized. It also helps to prevent hair follicle damage. Always protect your hair before you go to bed or rest your head on rough surfaces if you do this style. Drink enough water to enhance the steady supply of sebum that is needed to keep your hair moisturized.

This styling method is a way of finding out the state of your hair. If your hair uniformly and beautifully recoils back to its natural Afro length while it air-dries, that means it is healthy. If it recoils unevenly, with some hair strands not recoiling at all, then it means your hair is unhealthy.

How to Simply Style Short Afro Hair

- Wash and properly rinse off shampoo residues from your hair, as earlier directed. You do not have to put your hair in sections since it is still short.
- Apply your natural hair moisturizer to your hair by gently rubbing it in with your fingers.

- Next, use a wide-tooth comb to comb your hair in a row-like manner, combing from one row to another. This helps to keep your hair strands uniformed.

- Finally, use your fingers to gently even-out the tips of your hair strands and allow your hair to recoil to its natural length as it air-dries.

Additional Points

Whenever you do this hairstyle, always refreshen your hair by moisturizing and combing it from time to time. Use a hair spray bottle with water to moisturize your hair before you comb it. Comb and apply hair products to your hair in a row-like manner.

Run water through your hair while you comb it if you use the shower method. This helps make combing easier and to make your hair strands recoil evenly. Drink enough water to help keep your hair moisturized.

Do not stress your scalp by pulling your short hair in the process of styling it. Always wear your hair freely or do simple styles since your hair is still short. Be gentle on your scalp while styling to prevent any hair follicle damage that can impede hair growth. Avoid using hot irons or blow dryers to style your hair. They drastically weaken Afro hair shaft, and lead to hair thinning and breakage.

Styling Children's Afro Hair

If you are a parent or childcare provider, the children you take care of rely on you for haircare decisions. Try your best to make decisions that will not hurt children under your care. Be patient with them while styling their hair. Style their hair in a way that will not damage their hair follicles.

Do not braid, thread, or relax children's hair. Their scalps are still tender, and their brains are still developing. They do not need to deal with the pain and complications that come with these hairstyles. Their hairstyles should not distract them from learning at school. Do not do their hair with beads or other hair accessories that will be heavy for their heads.

Their hairstyles should be simple and loose. You can either wash, moisturize, comb, and let them wear their hair freely with no hair bands, or hold their hair in one, two, or three loose sections.

Be very gentle when combing their hair. Always comb their hair with a wide-tooth comb, and make sure their hair is well moisturized before combing.

Chapter Five

Hair Damaging Contacts

Whatever your hair consistently rubs against can either strengthen or be harmful to it. Your hair rubs on different surfaces daily, like your bed headboard, car seat headrest, walls, bed linen, and more. Instead of letting your hair directly rub against rough surfaces that can cause damage to it, cover it with a scarf or hair cover made with a soft fabric like silk.

Silk fabrics are good for Afro hair. Silk is a natural protein derived from cocoons of insect larvae and knitted into fabrics. Good quality silk fabrics are breathable, and they help reduce hair damage when they are used to make hair accessories and pillowcases. Silk also has anti-aging properties that help improve skin appearance. Silk fabrics make the skin feel soft and smooth after sleeping on bed linens made with them.

You can either use a silk scarf to cover your hair before bed or sleep on a silk pillowcase to help protect your hair. You can also use silk fabrics to make car headrest covers and couch pillow covers to help protect your hair from becoming dry when you rest your head on them.

Cotton and other fabrics that are not soft are not recommendable for Afro hair. They do not protect Afro hair or help retain hair moisture like silk fabrics do. They absorb natural oils from the hair, which leads to hair frizz and dryness. Afro hair strands also have a way of coiling into cotton fabrics when you sleep on cotton pillowcases. This does not happen when you sleep on silk pillowcases as silk fabrics have smooth surfaces that allow your hair to glide through them with less friction. If you want to purchase a silk fabric for your hair accessories, be sure to buy 100% silk material because some of them are mixed with other types of fabrics.

It is important to note that silk fabrics fade with time, just like other fabrics. However, they can last longer if you take proper care of them. To care for your silk products, always hand-wash them with a non-toxic soap and allow them to air-dry. It does not take long for silk materials to dry. If you wash your silk pillowcase in the morning and let it air-dry, it should dry before your bedtime.

If you prefer to use washer and dryer, still use a soft and non-toxic soap to wash your silk products and dry them on cool setting. Silk fabrics are usually wrinkled after they air-dry. If you are concerned about this, you can iron your pillowcases on low heat to get back that smooth and soft feel for your comfort.

Wash your silk pillowcases regularly to prevent any kind of facial breakouts if you have a sensitive skin. The hair products you apply to your hair get on your pillowcase whenever you lay your head on your pillow. If the oily particles from the products stay on your pillowcase for too long, they can accumulate germs, which can eventually get transferred to your face and lead to skin breakouts.

If you prefer to cover your hair instead of the silk pillowcase option, you can cover it with a silk head cover before going to bed. This helps to reduce hair tangling, hair dryness and hair breakage.

Avoid wearing hair covers with elastic bands. It is uncomfortable to wear tight hair covers with elastic bands, especially when sleeping. They restrict blood flow to the regions of the head, which is one of the reasons most people wake up with swollen and pale faces when they wear them to sleep. Instead of an elastic band, you can have your hair cover or bonnet lined loosely around it with a silk fabric to help improve blood flow and protect the hair around your edges. You can get the ones with ties to help you control the way they fit around your head.

Do not use hair accessories that can potentially cause damage to your hair or hurt your scalp. Hair accessories like metal bobby pins with rough edges can gradually cut your hair if you use them consistently. Other metal hair accessories like hair clips and clip-ins should be avoided as well.

Do not use tight hair holders, or those that your hair strands can get tangled on, to hold your hair. Do not put your hair in tight styles. Putting your hair in tight styles can damage your hair follicles and lead to issues like baldness and skin rashes around your hairline.

Caps and hats are like wigs. The materials used in making them are rough on the hair and absorb natural oils from it. Most of them hold tight around the head, which can lead to the thinning of hair around hairlines. If you like wearing caps and hats, get the ones that can help keep your hair free from friction damage. You can line the parts that touches your hair with soft fabrics to help protect it.

Chapter Six

Sleep Well and Thrive

Sleep is so essential for our optimal health and well-being. It helps with rejuvenation and other systemic processes in the body. Sleep deprivation (the consistent lack of sleep) has detrimental effects on the body and hair. Some of the effects of lack of sleep that can directly or indirectly affect the hair include:

- Fatigue
- Headaches
- Memory issues
- Hormonal imbalance
- Immunosuppression

Hormones and Immune System

Sleep plays a huge role in balancing hormones in the body. Sleep deprivation disrupts this process and can lead to hormonal imbalance in the body, which can affect the hormones associated with hair growth and maintenance. Hormonal fluctuation can trigger hair disorders like premature hair graying, hair loss, baldness, stunted hair growth, brittle hair, hair dryness, and so on.

Sleep deprivation also has negative impacts on the immune system. It suppresses the immune system and makes it hard for the body to fight hair infections. If you have a hair follicle infection, but your immune system is weak due to lack of sleep, it will take longer for your body to overpower the foreign agents causing the infection. But if you are getting enough sleep to keep your immune system boosted, it will be easier to get rid of the infectious agents.

It is recommended for adults to get up to 7-9 hours of sleep per night and for children to get more hours of sleep, since it plays a huge role in their growth and development. This recommendation is not set-in stone. The amount of sleep adults need per night varies among individuals. Some people take less than seven hours of sleep per night, and are fully functional during the day, while other people need more than seven hours of sleep per night to make it through the day.

Did you know it takes longer for an injury a person sustains to heal when he or she is sleep deprived? Yes, find out for yourself. Compare the healing process of injuries you sustain when you are overly sleep deprived versus when you are getting enough sleep. If you are sensitive to the changes in your body, you will notice that the healing process is faster when you are getting enough sleep. If you are getting the hours of sleep that your body needs and making other healthy lifestyle choices, the healing of injuries you sustained in your hair or any of its related structures will not be delayed.

Good sleep is not just about the number of hours you slept (quantity), but how well you slept (quality). Good quality night's sleep entails that it is not hard for you to fall and stay asleep, you sleep soundly and wake up few times at night, and it is easy for you to fall right back to sleep after you wake up. Poor quality night's sleep is the opposite. In this case, it is difficult for you to fall and remain asleep, you wake up many times during the night and it is extremely hard to fall right back to sleep after you wake up. Poor quality sleep is a sleep problem that might not give the body enough time needed to complete its repair functions.

Avoid sleeping in a stuffy place. Always open your windows to ventilate your bedroom. If your bedroom gets stuffed with harmful substances and you continually inhale them, especially when you are sleeping, they can migrate to your hair or the structures related to it and cause damage to them. Even if they damage other structures that are not related to your hair, the signs can still show through your hair.

How to Improve the Quality of Your Sleep

- Create a convenient sleep schedule that can help you get enough sleep each night.

- Avoid sleeping with artificial light as that can affect your circadian rhythm, which regulates the sleep-wake cycle.

- End your screen time long before bedtime. If you really need to work on your phone while in bed, dim the screen light so it does not affect your ability to fall asleep when you are ready to sleep.

- Keep your devices away from your body, or turn them off before going to bed: your phone, tablet, computer, radio, etc. The electromagnetic waves that flow through them can negatively affect the quality of your sleep.

- Remove anything that can possibly obstruct your breathing, especially those with respirable harmful particles, from your bed before you go to sleep.

- Stay active during the day to help prepare your body to rest and sleep at night.

- Try not to take long naps during the day. Naps are good but keep them short.

- Sleep on slightly elevated pillow if you usually have gastroesophageal reflux or heartburn that interferes with your sleep.

- Completely stop the intake of alcohol, caffeine, and nicotine close to your bedtime, they can negatively affect your sleep.

- Keep your bed linens clean and think of other ways to make your bed and mattress more comfortable as that has significant impact on sleep quality.

- Write down your plans so you do not have to go over them repeatedly in your head, which can make it hard for you to fall asleep.
- Avoid taking sleep medications as they may have side effects that can negatively affect your sleep and hair.

Chapter Seven

What You Feed on Counts

The overall condition of your body mainly relies on what goes into it - be it food, water, medicine, herbs, alcohol, and so forth. Food nutrients are obtained from either animal or plant products, but plant products have higher nutritional values than animal products. Fruits and vegetables, most especially, are packed with nutrients that help improve hair growth. Plant products are easily digested and absorbed in the body better than animal products.

The foods we eat can get contaminated or adulterated before getting to our tables. Food contamination can occur accidentally or intentionally; however, food adulteration is deliberately initiated by people who handle or gain access to our foods before they get to us. It is crucial to know this because consistent consumption of polluted foods is extremely dangerous and has negative impacts on the hair.

The harmful agents in contaminated and adulterated foods can get in the bloodstream and migrate to different areas in the body. They can cause hair problems like hair dryness, hair loss, stunted hair growth, premature hair graying, and balding when they attack the hair or its related structures.

These agents can harm the body if the immune system is suppressed. If your body gets weakened by their harmful effects, it can negatively affect your ability and desire to take proper care of your hair. With this being the case, always check to ensure that the foods you eat are not contaminated or adulterated. You can grow your foods or buy them from farmers you trust to be on the safer side.

Processed foods, which are foods that are altered through different techniques during preparation, also have negative effects on the hair. They are usually canned, dried, frozen, baked, or pasteurized. They contain preservatives that are harmful, so try as much as you can to reduce or completely stop eating them. It is safer to prepare your food by yourself to avoid exposing your body to the preservatives and other harmful substances in processed ones.

Always consider the nutritional benefits of any food you intend to eat before you put it in your mouth. You should not just eat to have something in your stomach, but to keep your body nourished. Eating healthy is not as expensive as some people think. The same amount of money used to buy heavily processed foods can be used to buy healthy foods that can help improve the growth and health of your hair. It is about making sacrifices - giving up unhealthy foods for the ones you need to keep your hair and entire body strong.

When your body gets the right nutrients from the healthy foods you eat, that enhances its ability to produce strong hair with vibrant color. The factors that can hinder this from happening are ongoing ailments in your body or inconsistencies with applying other healthy haircare tips. These two factors can restrict your hair from thriving even when your body is getting the right nutrients.

The state of your hair is usually a physical indicator of what is going on inside your body. When something bad is happening inside your body, it usually shows in your hair.

The signs can show through hair discoloration, hair loss, hair breakage, hair dryness, and more.

If you have always maintained healthy hair, and it suddenly becomes the opposite, without anything changing in your haircare routine, something might be going wrong inside your body. In a case like this, try to see a doctor for proper checkup to prevent the issue from getting worse.

Genetically Modified and Organic Foods

It is not easy to get foods that are safe for consumption these days. As if food contamination and adulteration were not enough, genetically modified foods (GMOs) joined the list. GMO foods are plant and animal products that have had their genetic materials changed using technologies that modify and transfer genetic features from an organism to another. The technicians behind these modifications claim they do this to reduce crop loss, improve crop yield and enhance food appearance.

GMO foods are harmful. We expose our bodies to different kinds of harmful materials and substances from eating them. The modification also reduces the nutritional values of food. To get enough amount of nutrients to keep your body and hair healthy, always go for organic foods that are not genetically modified.

Organic foods are products such as fruits, vegetables, grains, dairy, and meats grown and preserved without any unsafe or chemical materials. Although most foods labeled as organics are not 100% organic, there is still a significant difference between them and conventional foods.

Make efforts to master the real taste and smell of the foods you eat. If any food you bought as organic taste or smell weird, that might be a clear sign that it is not organic, or it has been polluted. Some of the signs and symptoms you can have after eating contaminated foods include:

- Diarrhea
- Headaches
- Constipation
- Hair loss, hair dryness, and hair discoloration
- Abnormal or loud movements in the stomach after eating.
- Sudden changes in the body - skin rashes, joint pains, etc.
- Abnormal constituents in waste products - blood in stool or urine, abnormal urine color, abnormal stool shapes and sizes, etc.

Always consider these factors as you eat daily since only safe foods can immensely nourish your body to keep your hair healthy. Eat foods that undoubtably make your body feel the healthiest. Mainly those that are rich in protein and vitamins. Avoid starchy and high fat content foods, and ensure you are getting the right nutrients from the right sources.

Wash your food stuffs properly before you eat or cook them. Wash your fruits and vegetables multiple times since they are foods you can eat raw. For additional safety, always peel the skin of peelable fruits and vegetable before eating them. Wash them before and after peeling to eliminate reasonable amounts of contaminants in them.

Most of the problems, sicknesses, and diseases that affect our bodies arise from the foods and other things we ingest. Harmful substances in foods can target different structures in the body and cause damage to them. If they make their way to a person's hair follicles, for example, the person will start experiencing hair problems that he or she may never know originated from eating a contaminated food.

Keep your food preparation methods simple. Avoid processed spices and use natural ones to cook. Bad spices from foods you eat can literally block the free flow of good natural elements that your body releases (like sebum that is supposed to help protect your hair) from getting to your hair. Bad food spices can also move through your pores to your hair strands and weaken or discolor them.

Avoid eating foods that are not prepared in a healthy way - fried foods, partially cooked meats and poultry, etc. The side effects associated with eating them can directly or indirectly damage your hair. It is advisable to steam, boil, bake, stew, or roast your foods.

Make fresh juices from fruits & vegetables or drink water instead of drinking carbonated drinks and unhealthy beverages. Try not to follow the trend of blending different fruits and vegetables together. The food mixture confuses the body during digestion. The digestive system must work extra hard to sort-out the mixed foods for proper digestion and absorption to take place. Just wash and chop your fruits and vegetables in preferable sizes and eat. This way, your digestive system can easily identify and digest them.

When your body carries out its functions without delays, it helps keep things going. Your hair follicles, for example, will quickly get all they need to enhance hair growth and sebum supply.

Medications and Treatments

Most medications and medical treatments lead to serious damage to the hair. A treatment originally administered to target a problem in the body can reverse and go against the hair. Be mindful of the types of medications and medical treatments you receive. Do you really need them? Are there healthier ways to cure or manage the medical issue you have? These are some of the questions you need to ask yourself or your doctor before considering treatments that can potentially damage your hair.

Hair growth enhancement medications are not safe for your hair. You should also avoid them. Human digestive system does not digest medications. They accumulate in the body and can lead to health problems worse than the ones they were formulated to cure. Most people who take hair growth medications experience side effects like hair loss, hair thinning, and hair discoloration. Some of them end up cutting their hair when they can no longer deal with the outcomes.

Synthetic vitamins and supplements do not digest in our bodies as well. Avoid taking them as they are artificially made. You should be getting the vitamins your body needs from whole foods - legumes, grains, fruits and vegetables. Getting the right vitamins and nutrients from their natural sources enhances the rate at which your hair grows and stays healthy without any side effects.

Chapter Eight

Make Water Your Bestie

One of the fastest ways of naturally growing Afro hair is through drinking plenty of water. Drinking enough water daily increases the supply of sebum to Afro hair. This helps keep the hair strong and moisturized.

Dehydration, which occurs when the body does not have enough water to carry out its functions, is usually accompanied with inadequate supply of sebum. In most cases, insufficient sebum supply diminishes the vibrancy of Afro hair color, which can make a person's hair that is naturally black to look dusty brown.

Dehydration also leads to hair dryness. When you are dehydrated, your hair gradually dries out no matter the amount of moisturizer you apply to it. The hair dryness is usually stirred by different interrelated factors that include decrease in blood volume, poor circulation of blood, and insufficient supply of natural hair oils.

Other Indicators of Dehydration

- Dry lips
- Dry skin
- Headaches
- Constipation
- Concentrated urine

Whenever you notice any of these signs and symptoms of dehydration, increase your daily water intake. Drink clean water, not other liquids as they cannot substitute for water. If the signs and symptoms you noticed truly resulted from dehydration, they will gradually revert to normal after you rehydrate.

Drinking sufficient amounts of water daily also helps in neutralizing and eliminating foreign organisms out of the body. This process prevents hair related infections like folliculitis, ringworm, and so on. The three main ways your body can become vulnerable to infections include:

A. If you are immunocompromised.
B. If there is a wound on your skin with less protective barrier to stop foreign agents from getting into your body.
C. If the foreign organisms finally get into your body in enormous amounts.

You need to be aware of these three main factors to have a better idea of how to combat infections. You also need to always secure other portals of entry in your body to prevent foreign organisms from getting in through them: your eyes, nose, ear, mouth, and genitourinary openings.

If you always take precautionary measures to keep your body from getting invaded by foreign organisms, it will be hard for you to fall sick. If the harmful agents end up getting inside your body, drinking lots of water will help eliminate them before they are able to harm you.

The amount of daily water intake needed to keep us hydrated varies for people. However, it is recommended for adult males to drink up to fifteen and half cups of water and for adult females to drink up to eleven and half cups of water per day.

If you do not know the daily amount of water you need to be drinking yet, you can find out by slowly increasing your water intake daily and noting the amount that helps keep your hair and skin moisturized. The amount of water that undeniably makes you feel hydrated, should be about the approximate amount you need daily - this holds true for children as well.

It is important to always drink clean water. Drinking unclean water is almost as bad as being dehydrated since the harmful elements in the water can get in the body and stir up issues. The issues foreign organisms trigger in the body are among the main factors that worsen Afro hair problems - hair dryness, hair loss, hair breakage, stunted hair growth, etc. Do not drink, cook, or brush your teeth with water that is treated with chemicals. As explained earlier, these chemicals can predispose the body to serious hair and health problems.

Bear in mind that you can drink enough water that is supposed to help keep you hydrated and other disruptive elements will completely drain it from your body and bring you to a dehydrated state. The electromagnetic waves from technological devices and the electrical current that passes through them when they are being charged have a way of draining the body to a state of dehydration. Be very mindful of how you let your body get exposed to these devices.

Frequent urination triggered by infection can also keep you dehydrated even when you are drinking enough water. If this happens to you, reduce your water intake a little bit to cut down on the frequent urination. In addition to that, eat more of fruits and vegetables so your body can get well-nourished to fight the foreign organisms. When you feel better, you can get back to your normal daily water intake.

How to Improve Your Daily Water Intake

- Do not drink too much water at once. Drink a cup or take few sips at a time so your body can gradually absorb it. It is okay to drink plenty of water early in the morning before eating to help trigger a bowel movement, but drink at intervals throughout the day.

- Drink from water containers or cups you really like to encourage you to drink more.

- Measure and take note of the approximate daily amount of water that keeps you in the best shape and stick to that amount, so you do not over drink. In other words, stick to the amount of water that protects you from having dry skin, dry hair, dry lips, concentrated urine, and headaches.

- Stay active - run, walk, do household chores and your body will naturally thirst for water.

Chapter Nine

Stress-Proof to Protect Your Hair

Stress is the body's response to life experiences. It can be a positive or negative feedback depending on its duration. Short-term or acute stress is not bad and goes away quickly. It makes you aware of a sudden danger so you can keep away from the source of it. Stress becomes a problem when it lasts longer than weeks. Divorce, financial hardship, the death of a loved one, and difficult jobs are some of the life challenges that can make a person experience long-term stress.

Long-term or chronic stress can directly or indirectly affect your hair and lead to serious hair problems if not effectively managed. When the body is stressed, it releases hormones to help us deal with the stressful situation. The release of hormones associated with stress can sometimes take the wrong turn when things get a little out of control. This often leads to hormonal imbalance, which can lead to hair loss, hair thinning, balding, premature gray hair, and other serious complications that include:

A. Telogen effluvium – in this condition, it is believed that stress restricts the hair follicles from producing new hair strands.

B. Alopecia areata – in this condition, it is believed that stress causes the immune system to attack the hair follicles resulting to hair loss and hair thinning.

C. Trichotillomania – in this condition, it is believed that stress makes the patients to have strong desires to pull strands of hair from their scalps and other parts of their bodies.

The explanations above might not necessarily be what lead to these hair disorders, but the main point is that stress makes the body vulnerable, which in turn gives the actual causal agents the opportunity to stir them. Besides stress, the consumption of unhealthy foods and high exposure to toxic substances can lead to these hair problems.

The challenges that come with the hair issues listed above can make the people facing them to lose interest in taking proper care of their hair. They can also make them gravitate toward doing unsafe hairstyles to hide their hair. These are reasons it is important to learn efficient ways of dealing with stressors that are posing threats to your life.

Thinking about your plans or the challenges you are facing repeatedly is a form of mental stress. It really weighs the body down and may have a connection with premature hair graying. Premature hair graying can discourage most people from growing their natural hair without dying or covering it with wigs.

Stress can also make us neglect our looks or haircare routines. It can make us ignore washing our hair regularly, sleep little or too much, eat unhealthy foods, or drink less water. If you find yourself in a difficult life situation that hinders you from giving your hair the care that it needs, put your hair in a loose protective style and drink enough water daily to help keep it moisturized and reduce hair breakage. You can do loose two strand twists or any other protective style that works best for you.

Other Effects of Stress

- Weak immune system
- Headaches
- Insomnia - difficulty falling and staying asleep.

Stress suppresses the immune system, which weighs down the body's defense capabilities. You need your immune system to be active and in great shape when trying to grow your hair. Hair disorders like telogen effluvium, alopecia areata, trichotillomania, and other hair issues need the help of a strong immune system to get corrected.

How to Manage Stress Better

- Be intentional about the steps you take while going through a stressful situation, so you do not add more stressors to the existing ones. If it means staying away from people or jobs that add stress to your life, do it until you fully recover and are in a better state to either return to them or completely stay away from them.
- Thinking about the things that are stressing you doubles the stress, so find a way to intentionally

divert your mind to those things that make you feel good and happy.

- If you need to make plans toward a goal, write them down so you do not forget or over work your brain to remember them.
- Set attainable goals.
- If financial problem is the source of your stress, cut out the things you cannot afford and use your money wisely.
- Be positive. Believe that you will be fine and hang around people who support and encourage you.
- Engage in healthy activities that help your body relax.
- Have fun and meaningful conversations with playful people around you. You can make jokes out of the stressful situations you are facing and laugh about them. This will help put you in a good mood. Do not make things too hard on yourself.
- Avoid drinking alcohol or smoking to deal with stress. They will only make you go in cycles and still bring you right back to the initial problem.
- Adjust your haircare routine or start a new one to fit your current daily schedule.

If you practice these stress management tips or figure out other ways to effectively manage stress, it will make things way easier for you. It will not feel burdensome to keep up with your haircare routine when you are going through situations that are supposed to cause you stress. In other words, you will be able to keep whatever is trying to stress you out under control and still have the desire to take good care of your hair and entire body.

Chapter Ten

Observe and Self-Experiment

One of the ways to figure the reasons to strange changes in your body is through conducting a self-experiment. Self-experimentation is an experiment that one can conduct on him/herself. Most researchers use this method in their studies when they do not need a broad sample of research participants. You can use it at any point to find out what leads to sudden changes in your body without the aid of a specialist.

Self-experimentation is a great tool to use if you are in a position where you need to find out the effects of foods or hair products you use. It is not hard to conduct; in most cases, a lot of resources are not needed to complete the test.

You just need to observe a change in your body, ask yourself questions as to why you are noticing that change, and then come up with possible reasons that might have triggered the change. After that, repeat whatever you did with the possible triggers before the change occurred to pinpoint the actual one stirring up the issue.

Remember, when your body is not comfortable with anything it gets exposed to, it finds a way to show signals. It can take minutes, hours, or days for you to feel the signals depending on how sensitive you are to changes in your body. When you keep getting the signals but do not know the reasons behind them, conduct a self-experimentation to find out what your body is trying to tell you.

To carry out a successful self-experiment, you need to write out the possible factors that caused the issues you are concerned about, which are things you did or got exposed to prior to noticing the unwanted changes. For example, if you noticed that your hair feels super dry and want to find out what is causing it, list out all you did prior to observing the hair dryness and redo them again:

a) What you ate, including medications and drinks.
b) The products you applied to your hair.

c) What your hair rubbed against - fabrics, walls, hair accessories, etc.

You can complete the experiment in days or weeks depending on how long it will take you to redo the things you listed. During the test, make sure you record everything you did and the changes you observe. For each day of your experiment, skip doing one thing on the list and record the changes you observe at the end of the day. After that, analyze all you have recorded to check for any significant change that indicates the cause of the hair dryness.

There is a sample of self-experimentation after this chapter. You can go through it to help you understand the concept better. Feel free to build on what you learned to conduct other forms of self-experiments. That way, you can stop haircare practices that are not useful and improve on those that are beneficial to your hair. There are "Root Cause Analysis" flowcharts after the self-experimentation sample that you can also refer to for quick solutions to common Afro hair problems.

Try as much as you can to always apply all the hair and health care tips shared in the previous chapters. Keep away from anything that tries to tempt you to denature your Afro hair or use other harmful haircare techniques.

All the haircare tips shared in this book work hand in hand. The hair is usually affected if any of them is neglected for a long period of time. If you are making enough effort to keep your hair clean and moisturized, you also must ensure you are doing the right hairstyles, protecting your hair, getting enough sleep, eating healthy, managing stress the right way, and drinking enough water to maintain healthy hair.

Let us keep encouraging each other and not relent in sharing valid haircare tips, especially with younger people and those who are seriously struggling with caring for their Afro hair. By doing this, we can gradually progress to a point where afro haircare challenges, the societal pressures to mask Afro hair with artificial hairs, and harmful Afro haircare practices will be history.

Self-Experimentation Sample

Kelly noticed that her hair feels so dry most times and was observably dry a day before her birthday. Prior to noticing the change, she did all that are listed below:

a) Had fruit salad for breakfast, lentils for lunch, and a bowl of fish soup for dinner.

b) Applied olive oil and brand-A oil she bought from a nearby store to her hair.

c) Took a nap after lunch on a silk pillowcase.

She does not think the hair dryness is linked to dehydration because she drinks enough water daily. For this reason, she marked dehydration off as a possible cause of her hair dryness. After listing the possible factors causing the hair dryness, she decided to conduct a self-experiment the coming week, starting from Sunday to Friday. The week approached and she started the experiment.

On the first day (Sunday), she had fruit salad for breakfast, lentils for lunch & dinner, applied olive oil and brand-A oil to her hair, took a nap after lunch on a silk pillowcase, and excluded eating a bowl of fish soup.

The second day (Monday), she had fruit salad for breakfast and lunch, a bowl of fish soup for dinner, applied olive oil and brand-A oil to her hair, took a nap after lunch on a silk pillowcase, and excluded eating lentils.

The third day (Tuesday), she had lentils for breakfast and lunch, a bowl of fish soup for dinner, applied olive oil and brand -A oil to her hair, took a nap after lunch on a silk pillowcase, and excluded eating fruit salad.

The fourth day (Wednesday), she had fruit salad for breakfast, lentils for lunch, a bowl of fish soup for dinner, applied only olive oil to her hair, took a nap after lunch on a silk pillowcase, and excluded applying brand-A oil to her hair.

The fifth day (Thursday), she had fruit salad for breakfast, lentils for lunch, a bowl of fish soup for dinner, applied brand-A oil only to her hair, took a nap after lunch on a silk pillowcase, and excluded applying olive oil to her hair.

The sixth day (Friday), she had fruit salad for breakfast, lentils for lunch, a bowl of fish soup for dinner, applied olive oil and brand-A oil to her hair, and excluded letting her hair touch any fabric during the day.

She recorded all she did, went through them after the experiment, and found out that Wednesday was the only day that her hair retained moisture. She went over her notes again and confirmed that Wednesday was the day she excluded applying brand-A oil. She quickly noted that applying brand-A oil might be the cause of her hair dryness since her hair stayed moisturized when she did not apply it.

She repeated the experiment and still had the same result. Then she finally admitted that brand-A oil is not suitable for her hair. She stopped using it and noticed that her hair was retaining more moisture. She felt so happy to have figured the cause of her hair dryness through self-experimentation and decided to always use the method whenever she notices any alarming changes in her body.

Root Cause Analysis

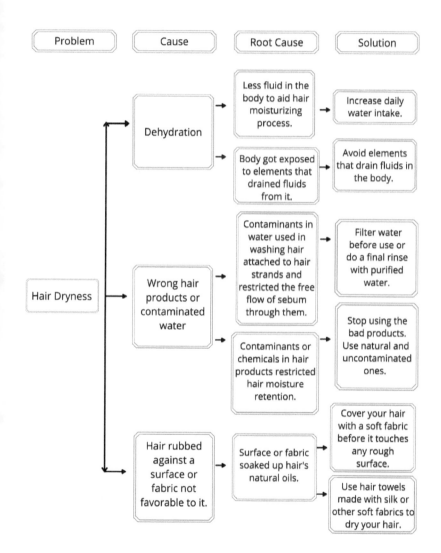

Problem	Cause	Root Cause	Solution
Hair Dryness	Dehydration	Less fluid in the body to aid hair moisturizing process.	Increase daily water intake.
		Body got exposed to elements that drained fluids from it.	Avoid elements that drain fluids in the body.
	Wrong hair products or contaminated water	Contaminants in water used in washing hair attached to hair strands and restricted the free flow of sebum through them.	Filter water before use or do a final rinse with purified water.
		Contaminants or chemicals in hair products restricted hair moisture retention.	Stop using the bad products. Use natural and uncontaminated ones.
	Hair rubbed against a surface or fabric not favorable to it.	Surface or fabric soaked up hair's natural oils.	Cover your hair with a soft fabric before it touches any rough surface.
			Use hair towels made with silk or other soft fabrics to dry your hair.

ROOT CAUSE ANALYSIS

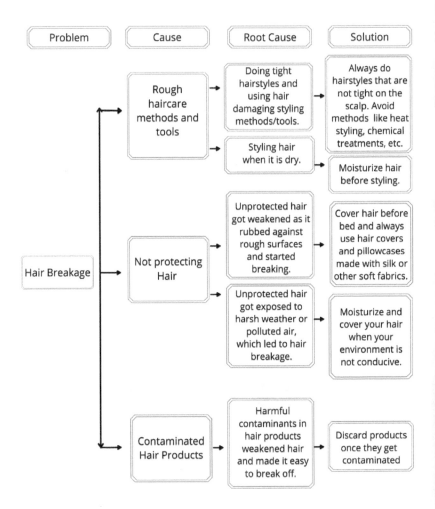

ROOT CAUSE ANALYSIS

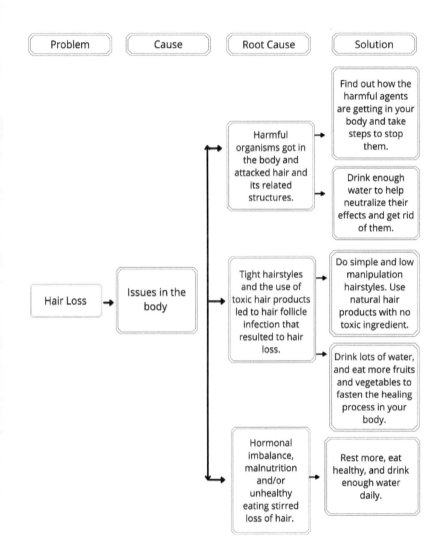

Problem	Cause	Root Cause	Solution
Hair Loss	Issues in the body	Harmful organisms got in the body and attacked hair and its related structures.	Find out how the harmful agents are getting in your body and take steps to stop them.
			Drink enough water to help neutralize their effects and get rid of them.
		Tight hairstyles and the use of toxic hair products led to hair follicle infection that resulted to hair loss.	Do simple and low manipulation hairstyles. Use natural hair products with no toxic ingredient.
			Drink lots of water, and eat more fruits and vegetables to fasten the healing process in your body.
		Hormonal imbalance, malnutrition and/or unhealthy eating stirred loss of hair.	Rest more, eat healthy, and drink enough water daily.

ROOT CAUSE ANALYSIS

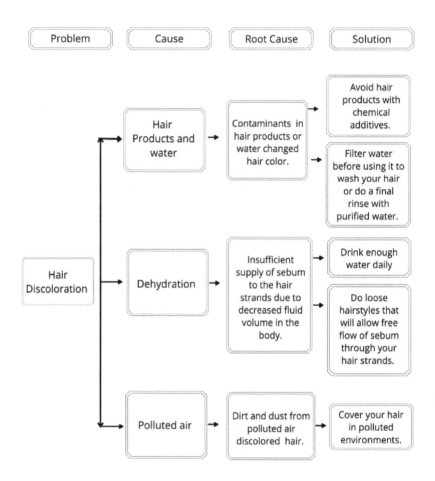

ROOT CAUSE ANALYSIS

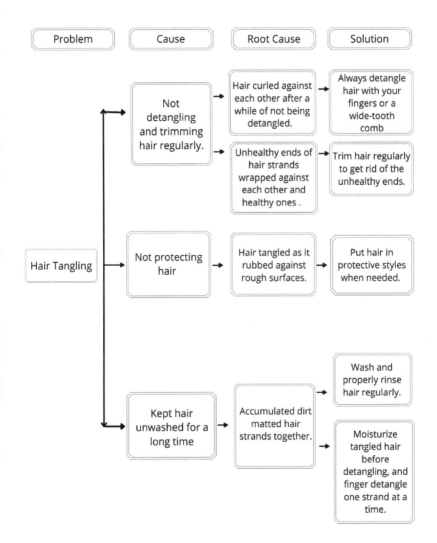

ROOT CAUSE ANALYSIS

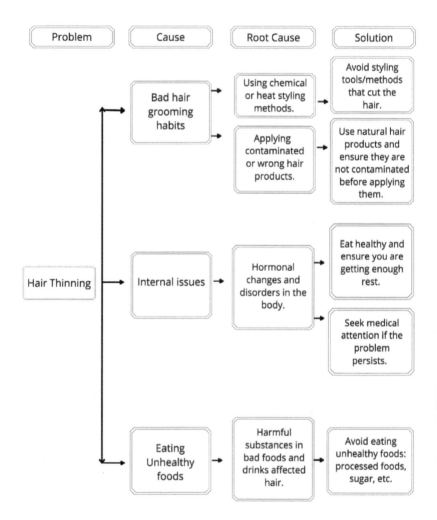

ROOT CAUSE ANALYSIS

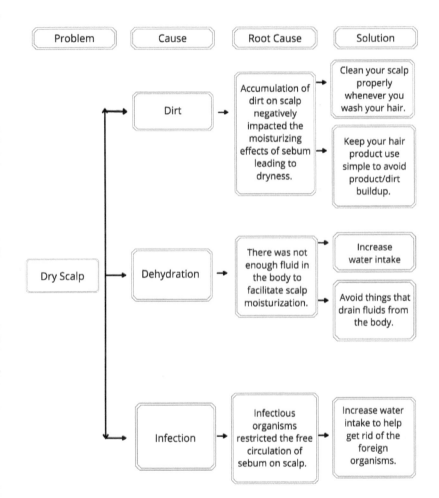

ROOT CAUSE ANALYSIS

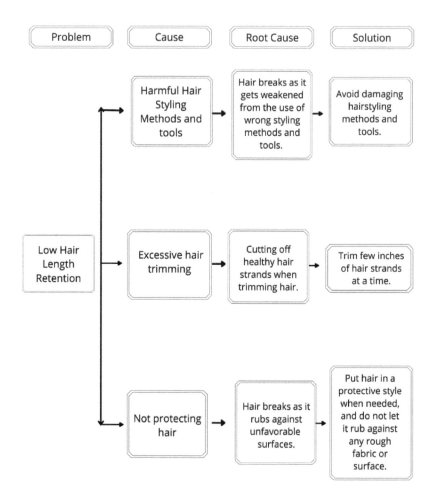

Problem	Cause	Root Cause	Solution
	Harmful Hair Styling Methods and tools	Hair breaks as it gets weakened from the use of wrong styling methods and tools.	Avoid damaging hairstyling methods and tools.
Low Hair Length Retention	Excessive hair trimming	Cutting off healthy hair strands when trimming hair.	Trim few inches of hair strands at a time.
	Not protecting hair	Hair breaks as it rubs against unfavorable surfaces.	Put hair in a protective style when needed, and do not let it rub against any rough fabric or surface.

ROOT CAUSE ANALYSIS

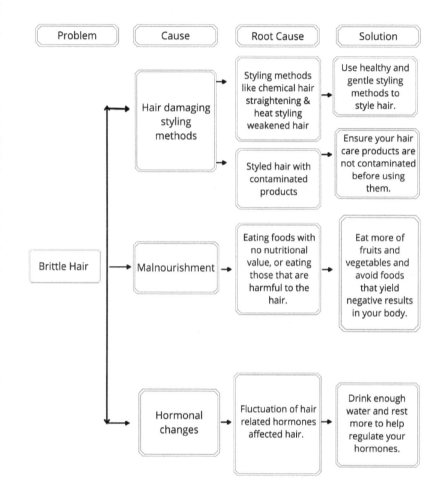

Problem	Cause	Root Cause	Solution
	Hair damaging styling methods	Styling methods like chemical hair straightening & heat styling weakened hair	Use healthy and gentle styling methods to style hair.
		Styled hair with contaminated products	Ensure your hair care products are not contaminated before using them.
Brittle Hair	Malnourishment	Eating foods with no nutritional value, or eating those that are harmful to the hair.	Eat more of fruits and vegetables and avoid foods that yield negative results in your body.
	Hormonal changes	Fluctuation of hair related hormones affected hair.	Drink enough water and rest more to help regulate your hormones.

ROOT CAUSE ANALYSIS

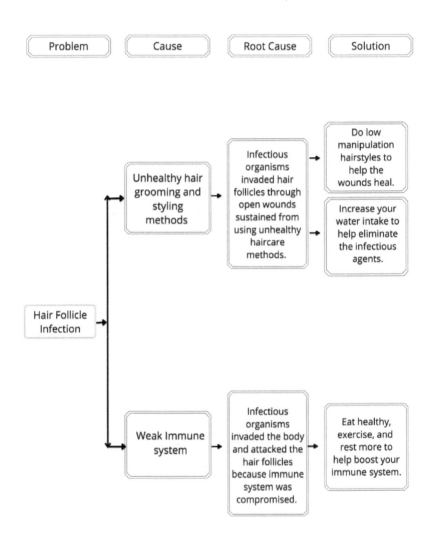

Problem	Cause	Root Cause	Solution

Hair Follicle Infection

Unhealthy hair grooming and styling methods

Infectious organisms invaded hair follicles through open wounds sustained from using unhealthy haircare methods.

Do low manipulation hairstyles to help the wounds heal.

Increase your water intake to help eliminate the infectious agents.

Weak Immune system

Infectious organisms invaded the body and attacked the hair follicles because immune system was compromised.

Eat healthy, exercise, and rest more to help boost your immune system.